Delivering the NHS Plan

next steps on investment
next steps on reform

Presented to Parliament by the
Secretary of State for Health
By Command of Her Majesty

April 2002

Cm 5503

£11.15

Contents

Executive Summary

1. There are two arguments that matter on the health service. One, how is it funded? Two, how is it run?

2. On the first question, more investment has to be paid for. Either through taxation, social insurance, or private insurance or individual charges. **No system is free.** Many systems are not only more expensive than taxation but leave millions uninsured, without any cover at all. We believe that the benefit of a universal tax based model is that it is an insurance policy with no "ifs" or "buts": whatever your illness, however long it lasts, you get cover as long as you need it. We made our choice in the Budget stating plainly that for the NHS to improve faster and tackle years of underfunding, more money is needed. The Budget now demonstrates how, within our tough public finance rules, **we will through general taxation be able to fund a 'catch-up' period to get us to health spending of 9.4% of GDP by 2008 – easily on a par with European levels of health spending**.

3. On the second question, we believe that any system for delivering health care must uphold the founding principle of the NHS – that it is free at the point of use based on need, not ability to pay. But Chapter 1 describes how **the 1948 model is simply inadequate for today's needs**. We are on a journey – begun with the NHS Plan – which represents nothing less than the replacement of an outdated system. We believe it is time to move beyond the 1940s monolithic topdown centralised NHS towards a devolved health service, offering wider choice and greater diversity bound together by common standards, tough inspection and NHS values. This will be underpinned by support for staff – with more staff, greater flexibility, increased

freedom to do their job even better. The aim: shorter waits, better cancer and heart treatment, modern but compassionate care.

4. So we believe in the traditional method of funding, but a completely new way of running the service. It is this **reform of the supply side** system design which this document focuses on.

5. Chapter 2 outlines some of the key benefits that this extra health spending will bring. **Waiting times for operations will fall from a maximum of 15 months now to 6 months by 2005, and 3 months by 2008**. Waits in A&Es and primary care will fall too. And extra investment in major conditions will cut cancer and cardiac death rates, and improve services such as mental health and for older people.

6. Chapter 3 summarises some of the key building blocks to growing capacity. Compared with latest available headcount figures, there are by 2008 likely to be net increases of at least **15,000 more GPs and consultants, 30,000 more therapists and scientists, and 35,000 more nurses, midwives and health visitors**. Primary care services will be expanded. More elective surgery will take place in new freestanding surgical units or 'diagnostic and treatment centres'. Hospital capacity is likely to grow by at least 10,000 more general and acute beds.

7. To help ensure that the large extra investment the NHS is now getting translates into capacity growth not inflation, **a greater share of the new funding will be used on training new health professionals for the future, and on capital infrastructure and modernised information technology rather than current spending**.

8. Chapter 4 explains that we are confident that the new national architecture we put in place in our first term is right. There is now broad support for a national body like NICE to ensure growing NHS spending is targeted on the most cost-effective treatments. There is wide support for National Service Frameworks covering cardiac, cancer, mental health services and other major conditions. There is consensus on the need for an external independent inspectorate to assure the quality of hospitals and primary care on behalf of patients. On the need to spread best practice through the NHS Modernisation Agency. And whereas the 1990s were spent debating internal NHS structures, there is now almost complete agreement that Primary Care Trusts are the right approach. So **in just five years, this new architecture has radically changed the way the NHS operates**.

9. But having got the structures right, Chapter 4 goes on to argue that we now need to introduce stronger **incentives** to ensure the extra cash produces improved performance. Primary Care Trusts will be free to purchase care from the most appropriate provider – be they public, private or voluntary. The hospital payment

system will switch to **payment by results** using a regional tariff system of the sort used in many other countries. To incentivise expansion of elective surgery so that waiting times fall, hospitals or DTC/surgical units that do more will gain more cash; those that do not, will not.

10. Chapter 5 underpins the new incentives with the introduction of **explicit patient choice**. Over the next four years, starting this year, the Scandinavian system will be progressively introduced across the NHS in which patients are given information on alternative providers, and are able to switch to hospitals that have shorter waits. By 2005 all patients and their GPs will be able to book appointments at both a time and a place that is convenient to the patient. This might include NHS hospitals locally or elsewhere, diagnostic and treatment centres, private hospitals or hospitals overseas.

11. Chapter 6 explains that as NHS capacity grows organically, we will continue to use private providers where they can genuinely supplement the capacity of the NHS – and provide value for money. This will also expand choice and **promote diversity in supply**, particularly for elective surgery. New PFI mechanisms, joint venture companies, and international providers will all be developed.

12. **Devolution** to the frontline will be stepped up, as Chapter 7 describes. The Department of Health will be slimmed down as, for example, in future negotiations over national employment contracts will be undertaken by NHS employers collectively rather than by the Department of Health. Instead of all public capital being allocated by the Department of Health from Whitehall, we will consider establishing an **arms-length Bank, controlled by the NHS itself**, which would invest capital from the Budget settlement for long term and innovative capacity growth and redesign. It will particularly focus on strategic shifts in configuration to more community and primary care based services. As regards revenue funding, locally run **Primary Care Trusts will hold over 75% of the growing NHS budget**.

13. The first NHS **foundation hospitals** will be identified later this year, with freedom and flexibility within the new NHS pay systems to reward staff appropriately, and with full control over all assets and retention of land sales. We will explore options to increase freedoms to access finance for capital investment under a prudential borrowing regime modelled on similar principles to those being developed for local government.

14. Chapter 8 makes the case for a **radically different relationship between health and social services**, particularly to improve care for older people. As the Wanless Report suggests, we will legislate to make local authorities responsible for the costs of hospital bed blocking. Rather than imposing structural reorganisation or nationally ringfenced budgets, this scheme means that social services departments will be

incentivised to use some of their large 6% real annual increases to stabilise the care home market and fund home care services for older people. There will be matching incentive changes on NHS hospitals to make them responsible for the costs of emergency readmissions, so as to ensure patients are not discharged prematurely.

15. As well as growing the numbers of health professionals, there need to be **fundamental changes in job design and work organisation**. Chapter 9 sets out how this requires new contracts for GPs, consultants, nurses and other staff. The new NHS pay system will allow greater allowance for regional cost of living differences, and free local employers to design new jobs breaking down traditional occupational demarcations. In seeking to expand the size of the healthcare workforce, a careful balance will be struck between the need to pay staff competitive rates in tight labour markets, and the need to ensure productivity gains on a par with the wider economy. Staff will be supported to continue life long learning.

16. Given UK health capacity constraints, there are difficult judgements on the speed of funding increases. Too slow, and we miss the opportunity to improve the nation's healthcare, with the risk that people simply give up on the NHS. Too fast, and investment might produce input price inflation, rather than improved output and responsiveness. On best advice the Government has decided that 7.5% is the optimal level of real NHS growth in England over the next five years. Higher than that would be unlikely to expand healthcare capacity any faster. Lower than that would mean an excessive and growing gap between supply and demand. But the **Government is determined to ensure that additional funding is backed by independent oversight of how the resources are being used**, to ensure they deliver the intended results.

17. Chapter 10 therefore describes how at a local level, **PCTs will be required to publish prospectuses**, accounting to their local residents for their spending decisions, the range and quality of services, and explaining the increasing choices that patients will have.

18. At a national level, legislation will be introduced to establish a **new tough independent healthcare regulator/inspectorate** covering both the NHS and the private sector, with a new Chief Inspector of Healthcare – not appointed by Ministers and reporting annually to Parliament. An equivalent body will be created for social services.

19. In summary the NHS is now on a stable financial footing and can face the future with confidence: with the NHS Plan in place; investment and reforms beginning to show results; power shifting to the NHS frontline. The changes will take time. But with investment to reform, the best days of the NHS are ahead of us, not behind.

1948 model	New model
Values: free at point of need	**Values:** free at point of need
Spending: annual lottery	**Spending:** planned for 3/5 years
National standards: none	**National Standards:** NICE, NSFs and single independent healthcare inspectorate/regulator
Providers: Monopoly	**Providers:** Plurality – state/private/voluntary
Staff: rigid professional demarcations	**Staff:** modernised flexible professions benefiting patients
Patients: handed down treatment	**Patients:** choice of where and when get treatment
System: top down	**System:** led by frontline – devolved to primary care
Appointments: long waits	**Appointments:** short waits, booked appointments

1

Investment + reform = results

1.1 The NHS Plan is the Government's ten year programme of investment and reform. It was drawn up in co-operation with NHS staff and patients. The NHS Plan principles were endorsed by leading professional and patient organisations. The evidence now shows the NHS Plan is working.

1.2 The NHS Plan will deliver for the people of our country a health service fit for the twenty first century with services designed around the needs of patients and improved health outcomes particularly for the poorest in our society. The vision in the Plan is for prompt, convenient, high quality services which treat patients as partners. It is of a vision where staff are fairly treated, properly rewarded and are able to use their skills to the full.

1.3 To support this vision, the Plan set out a coherent framework of:

- high national standards and clear accountability;
- devolution of power and resources to the front line to give health professionals who deliver care the freedom to innovate;
- increased flexibility between services and between staff to cut across outdated organisational and professional barriers; and
- a greater diversity of service providers, and choice for consumers.

Progress to date

1.4 There has already been important progress towards an expanded and reformed NHS:

- while the effects of decades of underinvestment still take their toll on services and staff, expansion and improvement is underway. Health outcomes are improving with death rates from both cancer and heart disease down. Patients referred urgently with suspected cancer are being seen in two weeks by hospital specialists and the maximum wait for heart operations has been cut by one third. More patients are being treated in primary and secondary care with more of the latest drugs being available to patients regardless of where they live. Waiting times to be treated in hospital, to get an ambulance, or to see a family doctor are all falling. Delayed discharges from hospital are falling too. Staff numbers are rising. Investment in new equipment and a huge hospital building programme are beginning to deliver more modern facilities for patients. Wards are cleaner and food is better. The NHS is at first base on implementing the ten year NHS Plan;

- the Bristol Inquiry, the Government's response and new legislation have articulated more fully how patients will be put at the centre of the service and how the framework for high quality standards and accountability will operate. We are confident that the new standards architecture we have put in place is right. There is now broad support for a national body such as the National Institute for Clinical Excellence (NICE) to ensure growing NHS spending is targeted on the most cost effective treatments. There is wide support for National Service Frameworks covering cardiac, cancer, mental health services and other major conditions. There is consensus about the need for effective regulation, inspection and quality assurance of health care in our country, arms-length from the Department of Health. With the National Patient Safety Agency and the NHS Modernisation Agency there are now new systems for when things go wrong and more help to learn from what goes right. So, in just five years, this new national architecture has radically changed the way the NHS operates;

- reforms are beginning to bite. Services are being redesigned as barriers between health and social care start to be broken down. Working practices are beginning to change as arbitrary demarcations between staff are eroded and more frontline staff are given greater authority. Star-ratings of hospitals are beginning to enable greater freedoms to be enjoyed by the best, whilst in a small minority of persistently poorly performers the management is being franchised. The NHS and the private sector are working together more closely than ever before. Tens of thousands of nurses are now able to prescribe drugs. Ward sisters are now in charge of ward budgets. Reforms led by staff in cancer services have cut waits and improved patients' experience. We have rolled out a programme of Patient Advice and Liaison Services across the NHS to provide advice and information to patients and help resolve problems on the spot;

- the old top down structure that has dominated the NHS for decades is beginning to give way to a new more decentralised approach. The old NHS Regional Offices and the health authorities have been abolished. Power is moving out of Whitehall. New Strategic Health Authorities (StHAs) are coming into being to oversee local health services. Primary Care Trusts are in place throughout the country already controlling half of the total NHS budget and soon to control 75% of it.

Funding growth for the long term

1.5 The NHS Plan is working. The Government is committed to its implementation as the cornerstone of our NHS reforms. The extra resources for the NHS and social services announced in the 2002 Budget now allow us go further in driving forward reform. The five and three year settlements for health and social care respectively allow both services to plan ahead with confidence and stability. For the NHS, there is an annual average increase of 7.5% above inflation over the five years 2003–04 to 2007–08. This is now the largest ever sustained increase in NHS funding, and exceeds the funding announced in the last spending review settlement (March 2000), when the NHS received annual average increases of 6.3% above inflation. It is also more than twice the annual average increase over the thirty year period from 1971 to 2001 (3.4%).

1.6 For personal social services (PSS) the Budget delivers annual average growth in real terms of 6% from 2003/04 to 2005/06. This demonstrates the Government's firm commitment to Social Care. In the last Spending Review, on a like for like basis, total PSS resources increased by an average of 3.3% in real terms over the three years (2001–2 to 2003–04). By comparison between 1992 and 1997 the average real terms increase was less than 0.5%.

1.7 These resources will be committed to building capacity to allow more patients to be treated and more people cared for more quickly and to higher standards. They will also be used to reform the way we use our existing capacity, allowing staff to work differently and reforming the way services are delivered. The biggest problem facing the NHS remains shortages of capacity in staff and beds. The stability provided by the 2002 Budget resources will allow the NHS and social services to plan increases in capacity with confidence. Inevitably this process will be evolutionary as it takes time to train and recruit staff just as much as it does to put up new buildings. Where there is other capacity that we can use for the benefit of NHS patients – in the private sector and by bringing in new providers from overseas for example – we will use it. Significant new investment in IT systems will drive change.

1.8 The scale and significance of this investment also demands that we address the remaining weaknesses of the NHS. The NHS today is not only the product of decades of under-investment, it is also a product of a lack of reform. The NHS has huge strengths – not least its ethos and its staff – but it has some profound and historic weaknesses:

- chronic capacity shortages;
- weak or perverse incentives that inhibit performance;
- an absence of explicit patient choice;
- lack of co-operation between public and private provision exacerbated by separate regulatory systems;
- a top-down, centralised system that inhibits local innovation;
- health and social care systems that work against each other when older people particularly need them to work together;
- out-dated working practices which have prevented a more rational design of services and deployment of staff;
- lack of attention to the rights and responsibilities of patients;
- weak local and national accountability.

1.9 To a greater or lesser extent, these are problems with which health care policy-makers are grappling the world over. Critics here argue that these weaknesses are unique to Britain and put the NHS beyond reform. It is certainly true that unless these weaknesses are addressed the NHS will not be able to deliver the patient-centred, responsive services people today rightly expect. Unless radical action is taken now the NHS will not gain maximum benefit from the high and sustained levels of investment it is now receiving.

1.10 We understand these structural weaknesses. There is more that we need to do to put into the hands of the caring professionals in the NHS the tools they need:

- making sure that we have the right incentives to deliver improvements with payments for results;
- breaking down the barriers between health and social care;
- providing greater autonomy for local organisations to take action on behalf of their local communities.

1.11 But this is also about making sure services are responsive to patients by:

- giving patients more information about services and more say in how they are best delivered;
- offering patients explicit choice;
- judging the success of local organisations in terms of patients' own responses and what they think of the services they receive.

1.12 And it is also about making sure the NHS achieves value for the tax payer, building on an already efficient system, to:

- improve productivity;
- introduce independent scrutiny and inspection;
- strengthen accountability to the public it serves and who pay for it.

1.13 So, large scale investment must be matched with fundamental reform if the country is to get the best from these extra resources. The Government's formula is: investment+reform = results. This document summarises the further steps now to be taken to deliver the NHS Plan.

1.14 It outlines *what* the public can expect to see in improved services as the Plan is implemented. It describes *how* these improvements will be secured. It *does not* set out a raft of new targets for the NHS.

2

Improving health services

2.1 The NHS Plan set out an ambitious programme to improve health services and health outcomes. A start has been made with reductions in waiting times and improvements in outcomes. The resources from the 2002 Budget allow this programme to be driven forward in the years to 2008.

2.2 Special effort will be focused on reducing waiting times for treatment since this is the public's principal concern about the NHS. The main improvements patients will see include:

- by 2005 a reduction in waiting times for an outpatient appointment to a maximum of 3 months;
- by 2005 a reduction in the maximum wait for a hospital operation to 6 months, then falling to a maximum of 3 months by 2008 (with an average wait of half this time);
- a reduction in maximum waiting times in A&E departments to 4 hours by 2004 with average waits reduced to 75 minutes. There will be further progressive reductions in this maximum waiting time;
- a reduction in waiting to see a GP so that by 2004 patients are seen within 48 hours or seen by another primary care professional within 24 hours.

2.3 Faster services will make for better health. Action will be focused where it can make most impact on improving health outcomes and tackling health inequalities. Our objective is to improve the nation's health and to improve the health of the poorest fastest. The main improvements will be in:

- reducing deaths from cancer by implementing the Cancer Plan's improvements to prevention and treatment services. By 2008 we estimate that thousands of lives each year will be saved as a consequence of extra investment and reforms in those services;

- reducing deaths from coronary heart disease by implementing the national service framework's improvement to prevention and treatment services. By 2008 we estimate that 25,000 lives will be saved each year as a consequence of extra investment and reform in those services;

- tackling suicide and improving mental health by implementing the national service framework. By 2008 every patient who needs it will have access to comprehensive community, hospital and primary mental health services with round the clock crisis resolution and assertive outreach services available to all who need them. Suicide rates will be down by one fifth;

- promoting the independence of older people by implementing the national service framework. By 2006 a further 100,000 people each year will be supported to live independently at home through extra intermediate and home care services.

2.4 New national service frameworks covering other groups of patients will be introduced during this period. There will be a greater focus on prevention and inequalities as with, for example, extended smoking cessation services and extra help to reduce rates of teenage pregnancy.

2.5 These improvements will make the NHS the fastest improving health care service in Europe. By 2007/8 UK health spending will reach 9.4% of GDP compared with the current EU average of around 8%.

2.6 None of this can be achieved unless every penny of the extra resources from the 2002 Budget is used wisely. That means focusing resources on securing the extra staff and facilities the NHS needs. It also means reforming how the NHS works.

2.7 Subsequent chapters describe the further steps on reform.

3

Expanding capacity

3.1 The funding increase announced in the Budget will enable us to take forward the next phase of the NHS Plan. It made commitments to substantial extra capacity in the health service – extra staff, new buildings, more beds, better IT and more new equipment. Since the Plan was published good progress has been made. For example, in just two years, the number of nurses has increased by over 20,000, achieving the NHS Plan target two years early. For the first time in 30 years there has been an increase in the number of general and acute beds in NHS hospitals.

3.2 Nonetheless the NHS still suffers from major capacity constraints. The extra resources provided by the 2002 Budget allow us to go further in tackling them. We will overcome the constraints through investment in staff and facilities and by doing things differently.

3.3 A deliberate element in our investment strategy for this spending review settlement is to ensure that a large share of the extra resource is used for medium and long term investment in capacity rather than for current spending. This will take the form of a step change in capital spending, higher investment in information and communications technologies, and the training of future health professionals.

3.4 We will recruit and retain increasing numbers of key staff using the extra investment announced in the Budget. By 2008 we expect the NHS to have net increases over the September 2001 staff census (latest available headcount figures) of at least:

- 15,000 consultants and GPs;
- 35,000 nurses, midwives and health visitors;
- 30,000 therapists and scientists.

3.5 Compared with 2001/02, by 2008 there will be over 8,000 more nurses each year leaving training – a 60% increase. Similarly, there will be an extra 1,900 medical school graduates per year – a 54% increase.

3.6 Hospital capacity across the system also needs to be expanded to enable people to get faster access to diagnosis and treatment and, in particular, to get waiting times down to a maximum of 3 months for inpatient treatment by 2008. The extra investment will allow us to plan for an increase in treatment capacity equivalent to over 10,000 beds. Existing NHS general and acute bed capacity currently stands at around 135,000 beds.

3.7 In addition we will expand and make better use of hospital capacity through a combination of measures. By 2008 we expect the NHS will have:

- increased the number of operations carried out as same day cases to over 75% of all operations – the equivalent of adding an extra 1,700 general and acute beds in hospitals;
- opened 42 additional major hospital schemes mostly delivered through the PFI with 13 more major schemes under construction;
- additional fully operational Diagnostic and Treatment Centres – the new generation of fast-track surgery centres which separate routine from emergency surgery.

3.8 The government's strategy is not simply to rely on expanding hospital capacity but to use the extra investment to modernise the way services are delivered in order to expand the choices available to patients. We will do this by:

- expanding the capacity of NHS Direct from 7.5 million callers per year to 30 million callers per year to provide advice, and direct patients to the most appropriate service for their needs. NHS Direct will, for example, handle all out of hours calls to GPs and will take up to 1 million low priority ambulance calls;
- increasing the amount of activity which takes place in primary and community settings with for example, millions more outpatient appointments taking place in the community rather than in hospital;
- establishing around 750 primary care one-stop centres across the country to offer a broader range of services, backed by more primary care nurses and specialist GPs, pharmacists, therapists and diagnostic services;

- extending intermediate, home care and residential care provision to offer alternatives to unnecessary hospital admissions and reduce delayed discharges. Extra social services resources will allow local authorities to increase care home fees where this is necessary to stabilise the care home market and increase choices for older people. We expect the expansion in intermediate care to increase provision by about 30% by 2005/6;
- electronic booking of appointments across the NHS by 2005 and electronic patient records in all PCTs and trusts by 2008.

3.9 Further details about the additional facilities and staff that will now become available following the Budget announcement will be published over forthcoming months.

3.10 To secure the best use of the resources, the reform programme outlined in the NHS Plan will now need to be driven forward. The chapters that follow describe further how this will happen.

4

Incentives for performance

4.1 The NHS Plan set out a new delivery system for the NHS with standards set nationally and greater devolution to deliver change locally. The system of earned autonomy outlined in the NHS Plan involves devolving more power and resources to frontline services as performance improves. The vision the NHS Plan aspired to was a move away from a top down centralised approach towards a more devolved health system with greater diversity and plurality of provision. The system would be held together by a common set of values, national standards and a tough system of inspection.

4.2 Since the NHS Plan was published:

- the NHS Modernisation Board has been established to oversee the implementation of the NHS Plan;
- new national standards have been published for cancer and older people's services;
- the Commission for Health Improvement (CHI) has completed over 100 reviews of local NHS services;
- the National Institute for Clinical Excellence (NICE) has helped to provide up to 1.5 million patients with up to £300 million worth of new drugs for conditions like cancer, heart disease, arthritis and alzheimers disease;
- the Modernisation Agency has been established and is already spreading best practice in service improvement;

- a new system of star rating for local NHS services has been introduced with accompanying action to give more freedoms to the best performers and intervention, including the franchising of management, in the poorest;
- appointments to NHS trust and health authority boards have been devolved from Ministers to an Independent Appointments Commission;
- Regional Offices and health authorities have been abolished with £100 million savings to be redeployed into enhanced childcare facilities for frontline staff;
- 302 Primary Care Trusts have been established to oversee the development of local health services and to control NHS budgets.

4.3 These structural changes are beginning to shift power and resources from the centre to the frontline in the NHS. Now the additional resources being made available will allow the NHS Plan's concept of earned autonomy to be taken forward.

Incentives for performance: introducing payment by results

4.4 In any health care system incentives shape performance. The history of the NHS is that it has had weak or perverse incentives and as a result has relied on top down instruction. This approach cannot work in a sector whose key asset is a professional workforce motivated by a desire to use their skills to improve care for patients. The right incentives will complement the commitment of the staff who want to treat more patients, to higher standards.

4.5 The NHS Plan commits us to the development of "a new system of incentives which will support the delivery of better services for patients." We have therefore carefully reviewed the way other countries structure their incentives. We have been careful to draw on lessons – both positive and negative – from these countries and from the internal market experiment in designing the new incentive mechanisms for the NHS.

4.6 At present there are no national financial mechanisms to support the movement of patients between providers (in the NHS or private sector) to support choice and make best use of capacity. For example, hospitals that are doing well in getting waiting times down are often forced not to use their spare capacity to treat more patients because that breaks through the budget ceilings they have been set. Conversely, poorer performers in the NHS are often bailed out with extra financial help. These perverse incentives need to be replaced with a new system that rewards good performers with more resources for appropriate treatment of more patients to higher standards.

4.7 We do not propose fundamental changes to the basic principle of allocating resources (on a needs basis) to PCTs who will then be free to purchase care from the most appropriate provider. Indeed the structure of UK primary care and the new unified budgets for PCTs create many rational and strong incentives at primary care level compared to other systems. They provide the correct incentives to take prevention seriously rather than merely expand the volume of hospital referrals.

4.8 In order to get the best from the extra resources we plan major changes to the way money flows around the NHS and differentiation between incentives for routine surgery and those for emergency admissions. Instead of block contracts for hospitals they will be paid for the elective activity they undertake. This is a system of payment by results. The reformed financial system will offer the right incentives to reward good performance, to support sustainable reductions in waiting times for patients and to make the best use of available capacity. Over time we will develop the system to improve the commissioning process by:

- providing patients with timely, comparable information on practices and hospitals updated regularly;
- offering choice to patients – choice of GPs, choice of hospitals and choice of consultants;
- ensuring that where choice is exercised cash for treatment goes with patients;
- setting the price for units of activity allowing the PCT to focus on volume, appropriateness and quality;
- offering commissioners and providers the flexibility to use savings and additional resources in a way that benefits staff and patients;
- requiring 'open book' relationships between PCTs and NHS Trusts.

4.9 We propose therefore to begin in the current financial year by testing different ways of moving resources with patients to establish the key principle that providers which fail to deliver lose money to those that can deliver. For 2003–4 we will introduce a regime under which:

- all providers will be contracted for a minimum volume of cases to achieve waiting time reductions;
- providers will lose money on a cost per case basis for failure to deliver;
- providers will earn extra resources on a cost per case basis for additional patients that move to them.

4.10 Experience of the internal market taught us that price competition did not work – particularly for emergency cases who were admitted to the nearest hospital – and merely led to excessive transaction costs. We will therefore use new Health Resource Group (HRG) benchmarks to establish a standard tariff for the same treatment regardless of provider. This is the hospital payment system used by many international health care systems.

4.11 There are a number of issues that we need to explore in more depth with the NHS as we develop this approach to ensure that adequate safeguards exist so that the system encourages appropriate activity growth. But these are matters that have been dealt with successfully in other countries and we shall learn from their experience.

4.12 In the medium term we propose to move to a system where all activity is commissioned against a standard tariff using either HRG or other appropriate measures. Local commissioning would focus on volume, appropriateness and quality, not price as this would be fixed using regional tariffs to reflect unavoidable differences in costs in different parts of the country. The more efficient providers would be able to retain some or all of any surplus they generated to deploy within their organisation to the benefit of patients and staff. The less efficient providers will be helped with support from the NHS Modernisation Agency to improve their performance. Where necessary new management could be brought in using the franchising process.

5

Choices for patients

5.1 The NHS Plan set out ambitious plans to create a health service that is more responsive to the citizens who pay for it and the patients who use it. A patient centred service demands more power for patients. The NHS Plan says "patient choice will be strengthened" and places particular emphasis on patient choice over hospital treatment including a choice over "a convenient date and time rather than being assigned a time by the hospital."

5.2 There are those who claim that a tax funded national system of health care can never deliver choice for patients. The example of Scandinavia proves those critics wrong. In Sweden and Denmark patients have access to information on waiting times and options for treatment, and patients who have been waiting for treatment have the choice of alternative provider.

5.3 From July this year the NHS will begin to offer similar information and similar choice to patients. We will start with patients with the most serious clinical conditions. From the summer patients who have been waiting six months for a heart operation will be able to choose from a range of alternative providers – be they public or private – who have capacity available to offer quicker treatment. We will also from this year move to publish on the internet and elsewhere regularly-updated information on waiting for all major treatments at all providers.

5.4 For the first time patients in the NHS will have a choice over when they are treated and where they are treated. The reforms we are making will mark an irreversible shift from the 1940s "take it or leave it" top down service. Hospitals will no longer choose patients. Patients will choose hospitals.

5.5 As capacity expands so choice will grow. We will roll out this new approach for other clinical conditions beginning in London later this year. We will do this carefully to maximise benefits both to patients and to taxpayers.

5.6 By 2005 all patients and their GPs will be able to book appointments at both a time and a place that is convenient to the patient. This might include NHS hospitals locally or elsewhere, diagnostic and treatment centres, private hospitals or even hospitals overseas. They will be able to compare different waiting times in different hospitals. By then the latest IT systems will allow GPs and patients to see which hospitals have capacity available to treat more patients more quickly and book on line.

5.7 Choice will be underpinned by new incentives. Those hospitals that have capacity to do so will earn more resources as the money follows the choice made by the patient. This is a sensible way of identifying and using spare capacity and, through the choices that patients make, providing new incentives for hospitals to treat more patients more quickly and to higher standards. In turn choice will create new incentives for hospitals not to build up long waiting times as they seek to expand activity.

5.8 Choice will also be underpinned by more information being provided to patients to help them make more informed choices. At a local level in each area the local PCT will provide independently-validated information to the public through its annual Patient Prospectus about the availability, the quality and the performance of local health services. The Prospectus will also contain details on the choice of services that are available in primary care – such as female GPs, or specialist services. At a national level the new Commission for Healthcare Audit and Inspection will provide detailed information not just on comparative NHS performance but on the outcomes of care that are achieved by different health services in different areas. Starting with mortality rates following heart surgery, this will include published information about outcomes by individual consultant teams.

5.9 For some services, for example emergency care, however, choice will have a more limited role to play. Here most patients will only want fast access to their nearest local hospital. For these services we will develop other mechanisms to ensure that local health services put proper weight on patient preferences. The star ratings that assess local NHS performance will, therefore, be linked to the scores that patients give, drawn from regular surveys of their views.

5.10 In turn, patient power will be backed by the new organisational arrangements we are making to put the voice of the patient at the heart of the NHS. There is further legislative change in the pipeline most notably to establish statutory independent

Patients Forums in each Trust, to monitor and review the quality of local services from a patient perspective, with one of their members elected to sit on the NHS Board.

5.11 These changes are all about shifting the balance of power towards patients in the NHS. These further steps will change the relationship between patients and services. Patients will be in the driving seat.

6

Plurality and diversity

6.1 The NHS Plan set out the framework for the NHS to "engage more constructively with the private sector." It made clear that ideological boundaries or institutional barriers should not stand in the way of better care for NHS patients. New partnerships needed to be developed so that the NHS could harness the capacity of private and voluntary providers to treat more NHS patients. But such partnerships would not compromise the fundamental principles underpinning the Plan: that healthcare should be available on the basis of need, not ability to pay. Any arrangements also need to be underpinned by high standards of care for patients and good value for money for taxpayers. And, above all, any capacity used in the private sector must augment, not subtract from, the number of precious skilled clinical staff already working in the NHS.

6.2 Since the NHS Plan was published:

- the Concordat between the NHS and the private sector has been published and has facilitated the treatment of thousands of additional NHS patients, enabling the NHS to help make progress on getting waiting times down;
- arrangements have been made to enable patients to be treated abroad through the NHS, with the first test bed schemes contracting for services with hospitals in France and Germany;
- the first arrangements for the private sector to provide diagnostic and treatment centres are under negotiation;
- the first clinical teams have been brought in from abroad in order to help boost NHS surgical capacity.

6.3 These developments will be reinforced over the next period of the NHS Plan. The extra resources made available in the 2002 Budget will secure a major expansion in NHS facilities. The historic deficits in capacity that bedevil the NHS mean that we will continue to use the private sector where it can genuinely supplement the capacity of the NHS and give value-for-money. This will promote diversity in provision of NHS services and increase the capacity that is available to NHS patients. There will be 5 further steps on reform here.

6.4 Firstly, we will extend the Private Finance Initiative (PFI) to other parts of the health and social care system. This will include substantial investment in new primary care facilities to support the increase in activity that we believe can take place there. There is also scope to upgrade mental health and community health and social care facilities by batching together smaller schemes into larger contracts. In the next phase of its development we will be looking to PFI to help support greater diversity of service provision to help shift the balance to community from hospital based care.

6.5 Secondly, PCTs and NHS Trusts will be able to use their legislative powers to form joint ventures with the private and voluntary sectors. They will for example be able to forge new alliances with housing associations to provide new forms of supported housing for vulnerable older people. They will also be able to enter into joint ventures with the private and voluntary sectors to provide NHS-supported nursing home accommodation. Again our intention is to forge alliances to promote more community based services to help extend patients' choices and to relieve pressures on hospitals.

6.6 Thirdly, we will develop new public private partnerships to support the rapid development of Diagnostic and Treatment Centres to help meet NHS waiting time reductions and provide more rapid, convenient and improved outpatient and diagnostic services in the community. The DTCs will help diversify service provision and, once again, relieve pressure on mainstream NHS hospitals.

6.7 Fourthly, we will maximise use of spare private sector hospital capacity backed by a new framework of prices based on HRGs within which contracts will be negotiated between PCTs, NHS Trusts and private providers. We estimate that up to 150,000 operations a year might be bought from the private sector for NHS patients.

6.8 Fifthly, recognising that the private health provider sector in England is relatively small, we will bring into the country overseas providers of health care – with their own clinical teams – to establish services for the NHS. These providers will either use existing NHS facilities where the NHS has spare physical capacity but cannot staff it or they will develop their own free-standing facilities which will often be DTCs. Given the recent interest in the "Kaiser model" of health care – in which greater investment in primary and community services produces short waits and good outcomes for patients – we will also encourage expressions of interest from successful international organisations to partner PCTs in developing and testing similar models of integrated care in the NHS.

6.9 These reforms will be underpinned by two further steps which are set out elsewhere in this document:

- first, the changes to the funding flows and incentives will support a greater choice for patients, improve efficiency and enable all providers – public or private – who offer good quality and value for money to more easily provide services for NHS patients;

- second, bringing together the different bodies with responsibility for inspecting and regulating health care will ensure consistent application of quality standards.

6.10 Together, these changes will ensure that the use of the private and voluntary sectors delivers both high standards of care to patients and good value for money for taxpayers.

7 Strengthening devolution

7.1 For fifty years the NHS has been subject to day-to-day running from Whitehall. A million strong service cannot be run in this way. If it is to better respond to the needs of patients the NHS can no longer be run as a monolithic, top-down, monopoly provider. Instead within a framework of clear national standards, subject to common inspection, power needs to be devolved to locally run services with the freedom to innovate and improve care for patients. The Government's aim, as the NHS Plan sets out, is for, "the centre to do only what it needs to do: then there will be maximum devolution of power to local doctors and other health professionals."

7.2 There will be a transition where more and more decisions about the NHS are taken locally rather than nationally. A start has been made with the abolition of the old NHS regional offices and almost 100 health authorities. As in any large organisation some functions will need to take place centrally. They will be strictly limited. The Department of Health will be slimmed down as power and resources are devolved out from Whitehall to the lowest level possible. In future, for example, we will move to a position where national negotiations over new contracts of employment will be undertaken by NHS employers collectively not by the Department of Health. Instead the Department will have the core functions of determining standards, distributing and accounting for resources and securing the integrity of the system through, for example, proper information and workforce planning.

7.3 The day to day management of the NHS will move to 28 new Strategic Health Authorities. They will become the local headquarters of the NHS. Their main functions will be to hold to account the local health service, build capacity and support performance improvement. Three-year franchises for running the StHAs will be let with performance judged against a published annual delivery contract with the Department of Health.

7.4 The real power and resources will move to the NHS frontline. Locally run Primary Care Trusts will hold the majority of the NHS budget. By 2004 they will control 75% of it. By 2008 we expect PCTs to control a larger share of the NHS budget. They will be free to commission care with decisions on providers increasingly informed by the choices which patients themselves make. This could be from primary care or hospital care, from a local NHS hospital or another NHS hospital, from the public, the private or the voluntary sectors. The PCTs will have freedom to decide where NHS resources are best spent including what to spend on their own clinical management infrastructure, but they will need to account publicly for how they have used resources against the test of high clinical standards and good value for money.

7.5 The NHS Plan set out proposals to give more freedoms to the best performing parts of the health service. It did so both as a reward for doing well and as an incentive for others to improve. Unlike the failed internal market experiment of the early 1990s we recognise that every hospital and every GP surgery needs to have the highest standards. Market structure in which most areas are served by only one or two local general hospitals means that competitive pressure alone is insufficient to guarantee high standards across all services for all patients. The stroke or heart attack patient is likely to be admitted to the nearest local A&E department come what may. That is why we have put in place new national standards, inspections systems and help to spread best practice. For the small minority of persistently poorly performing NHS organisations more help and support will need to be accompanied by more intervention. In these cases top performing trusts will be able to take over poorly performing trusts. Through the franchising process new management with a proven track record of success will be brought in.

7.6 Getting the right incentives in place can help raise standards everywhere. The new financial incentives set out in this document will help. But we also know from our discussions with people working in the NHS that the reward they most appreciate is having the freedom to get on and improve their local services to patients.

7.7 The first wave of three star trusts will be able to establish joint venture companies, get easier access to capital resources and will be subject to less monitoring and inspection. We have explored with them the scope to go further. These discussions led to the model of the "Foundation hospital" – fully part of the NHS but with greater independence than now. In other European countries similar models are commonplace and those hospitals have delivered impressive results for patients.

7.8 The first NHS Foundation Hospitals will be identified later this year. Foundation status will also be available to high performing Primary Care Trusts and Care Trusts as well as NHS Trusts. These Foundation trusts will have greater freedoms than existing trusts and will be able to use their freedoms to bring about benefits for patients.

7.9 Foundation trusts will have freedom to develop their board and governance structures to ensure more effective involvement of patients, staff, the local community and other key stakeholders. Foundation trusts will in this way reflect the spirit of public sector enterprise that our plans are designed to unleash.

7.10 Foundation trusts will operate to NHS standards, be subject to NHS inspection and abide by NHS principles. They will have the freedom and flexibility within the new NHS pay systems to reward staff appropriately. These will help promote diversity and encourage innovation.

7.11 The powers of foundation trusts will include full control over all assets and retention of land sales. We will explore options to increase freedoms to access finance for capital investment under a prudential borrowing regime modelled on similar principles to that being developed for local government.

7.12 Alongside this innovation on borrowing arrangements for Foundation trusts, we intend to reform the way public capital investment is undertaken in the NHS. We will consider establishing a new NHS body which will act as a bank for the NHS to replace the current informal system of brokerage whereby Trusts with a surplus of cash lend to Trusts that need it. That system has until now been managed from Whitehall by Department of Health civil servants. The NHS bank would instead be mutually controlled by the NHS and run by specialists in finance from the health service and elsewhere. The Bank would provide risk reserves for PCTs and overdraft finance for NHS Trusts. It would provide access to extra capital for long term and innovative investment from the extra capital resources for the NHS contained in the 2002 Budget settlement. By removing control from Whitehall we expect capital resources to be properly and fully utilised for the periods for which they are allocated.

8

Health and social services: one care system

8.1 Patients, particularly older people, need health and social services to work together. They rely on good integration between the two to deliver the care they need, when they need it. As the NHS Plan put it "if patients are to receive the best care then the old divisions between health and social care need to be overcome." Since the NHS Plan was published we have:

- begun implementation of the NSF for older people, by establishing a new single assessment process, converting Nightingale wards, and carrying out an audit of age discrimination;
- invested heavily in intermediate care to build a bridge between hospital and home for older people;
- reduced delayed discharges from hospitals with extra funding and improved local co-operation between the NHS and social services;
- increased the use of Health Act flexibilities through, for example, local pooling of health and social services budgets with £1 billion of investment now organised in this way;
- established the first Care Trusts to bring together in one local organisation health and social services, including older people's services;
- announced the introduction of star ratings for local social services performance and begun to introduce a new system of freedoms and rewards for the best performers alongside intervention for those with persistent problems.

8.2 The substantial increase in resources for social services – as well as for the NHS – calls for increased safeguards to ensure that the money is spent wisely and well. Our proposals for a toughened inspection regime will be crucial.

8.3 The substantial extra resources for social services will allow investment to take place in an extended range of services and to raise standards of care. Older people will be amongst the principal beneficiaries. Local authorities will be able to use the extra resources to stabilise the care home market and provide more care home places. In line with the NSF for older people, we intend for there to be a reducing reliance on institutionalised care in favour of more support for people to live independently. This will require expansion in intermediate care places – particularly to prevent hospital admission and to provide more rehabilitation – and in packages of home care. And there will be faster access to assessments and care.

8.4 These extra resources also provide the opportunity for further steps on reform towards the NHS Plan vision of a single care system which is organised in the interests of its users, not providers. Although progress has been made towards breaching the "Berlin Wall" between health and social care there are still too many parts of the country where a failure to co-operate means that older people fail to get the holistic services they need.

8.5 Older people are the single biggest users of the NHS. They are the generation which built and have supported the NHS all their lives. The commitment to deliver patient-centred care – the right care, in the right place, at the right time – must, above all, be honoured in the delivery of care for older people. And older people above all others have a right to expect that their care is delivered seamlessly through a range of services that are convenient and as close to home as possible.

8.6 New arrangements already being introduced for personal social services in 2002–03 will provide some of the framework for improvement with, for example, the introduction for the first time of a new £50m performance fund for intermediate care. But existing systems and incentives do not support co-operative working as well as they might.

8.7 Much of the recent progress on reducing delayed hospital discharge – so-called 'bed-blocking' – whilst welcome has been driven by top down targeting of resources, central intervention, and close monitoring of progress. But in the longer term this approach is not sustainable in a climate where the philosophy of devolution and earned autonomy is applied both in local government services and in health services.

8.8 Primary Care Trusts will help bridge the gap between hospital and community health provision but more needs to be done to bridge the even wider gap between health and social care provision. We know that health and social care staff want to see arrangements that more actively support joined up planning and provision of services. This is certainly what patients – especially older people – need to see.

8.9 We intend therefore to introduce new arrangements to ensure a more seamless services for patients. We will consult with local government on the implementation of these changes.

8.10 We have been impressed by the success of the system in countries like Sweden and Denmark in getting delayed discharges from hospitals down. We intend to legislate therefore to introduce a similar system of cross-charging. The new social services cash announced in the Budget includes resources to cover the cost of beds needlessly blocked in hospitals through delayed discharges. This was also a reform commended by the Wanless Review. Councils will need to use these extra resources to expand care at home and to ensure that all older people are able to leave hospital once their treatment is completed and it is safe for them to do so. If councils reduce the number of blocked beds, they will have freedom to use these resources to invest in alternative social care services. If they cannot meet the agreed time limit they will be charged by the local hospital for the costs it incurs in keeping older people in hospital unnecessarily. In this way there will be far stronger incentives in the system to ensure that patients do not have to experience long delays in their discharge from hospital. There will be matching incentive charges on NHS hospitals to make them responsible for the costs of emergency hospital readmissions, so as to ensure patients are not discharged prematurely.

8.11 We also intend to introduce other incentives to encourage use of the existing legal powers that local health and social services have to better integrate their services. The best performing trusts for example will be encouraged to use new powers to establish joint ventures to provide more seamless services for patients. We will also introduce further financial incentives to encourage the voluntary take-up of Care Trust status.

8.12 Finally, we will keep the relationship between health and social services under review. Older people and other service users have the right to expect that local services are working as one care system not two. We will monitor how far the NHS Plan and these further reforms we are proposing take us towards that goal. If more radical change is needed we will introduce it.

9
Changes for the workforce

9.1 NHS staff are our greatest asset and as the NHS Plan says, "NHS staff, at every level are the key to reform." We will never be able to achieve the modern NHS the nation needs without the active involvement of staff. This cannot be achieved by the traditional top-down management approach. Instead we intend to give frontline staff greater control over how local health services are delivered. This is at the heart of our reform programme.

9.2 To build the NHS our nation needs we will need to increase the number of staff. By itself however, employing new staff will not provide sufficient capacity to deliver the improvements we expect. Changes in working practices will be fundamental to delivering these improvements. In the way staff are employed and paid the NHS retains too many of its 1940s employment practices – overly demarcated and inflexible – and has learned too little from other model employers about the benefits of employment flexibility, linked to appropriate rewards and incentives. Flexibility cuts two ways: the NHS has to better support and involve staff in improving care for patients. Our objective is to liberate the talent and skills of all the workforce so that every patient gets the right care in the right place at the right time.

9.3 Over the last few years we have made progress towards this objective:

- negotiations are underway to reform the employment contract of family doctors and hospital consultants;
- negotiations are progressing on a new pay system for NHS staff through the Agenda for Change discussions;

- consultants have greater control over hospital equipment budgets, ward sisters have control over ward budgets and health visitors over community budgets;
- nearly 2000 modern matrons are in place with the clout to improve the fundamentals of care for patients in hospital;
- the roles of therapists and nurses have been enhanced through new consultant posts and new powers to prescribe drugs and treat patients;
- training and staff development opportunities are increasing and 90,000 staff are being supported to modernise services by the NHS Modernisation Agency;
- NHS employers are providing more opportunities for flexible working including better child care support.

9.4 The extra resources, provided by the 2002 Budget, will allow us to meet the NHS Plan's commitment to "liberating the potential of staff." Our further steps on reform will change working practices and help put frontline staff in charge of making improvements happen at all levels of the NHS.

9.5 We will modernise pay systems for all staff so that the right incentives are in place to break down demarcations and change working practices. We intend to press ahead with new contracts for GPs and hospital consultants. The aim here is to provide better rewards for those doctors making the biggest contribution to improving services for NHS patients. We also intend to introduce a new pay system for nurses and other NHS staff by concluding the Agenda for Change negotiations. Staff who take on new responsibilities and make the greatest contribution will get extra rewards. A fairer pay system will help recruit and retain more staff. The national job evaluation framework means that local employers will have local flexibility to pay staff according to the new roles they take on. Pay modernisation in this way will raise productivity and promote flexibility.

9.6 Reform of pay systems will help the NHS make optimum use of the talents of every member of staff. Pay modernisation will bring better career opportunities. It will also help provide the right incentives for staff to take on new responsibilities. We anticipate pay reform, combined with greater flexibility of roles and responsibilities could, with additional training and support, allow a growing share of the GP workload to transfer to nurses and other health professionals over the next three years; similarly, some of the consultant workload could transfer to other staff; as could some nurse and therapist workload transfer to support staff.

9.7 Every member of NHS staff eager to train will be entitled to individually-tailored professional development programmes through the new NHS University (NHSU). The NHSU will start work in 2003. It will begin by delivering common induction and communication skills for all NHS staff. There will be innovative common learning programmes across professions both pre-and post registration. Lifelong learning for the whole workforce will support staff to extend their skills and knowledge and take on new roles and responsibilities. Through the new Postgraduate Medical Education and Training Board for the first time the NHS, working with the Medical Royal Colleges, will be able to better balance the training needs of future doctors with the service needs of local communities.

9.8 To get the best from all NHS staff the health service needs to become a better employer. In future the 'star rating' performance assessments will include measures of how well each NHS organisation is supporting and involving its staff. There will be additional investment in flexible working, childcare support and personal development to underpin our programmes of recruitment and retention. An additional £100m will be invested in childcare by 2004 including providing childcare support for healthcare students.

10

Strengthening accountability

10.1 The extra resources provided by the 2002 Budget need to be backed by new mechanisms to ensure that the public gets the best value for money. Overall the NHS is an efficient as well as a fair way of providing health care. But it can be more efficient still which is why we expect to see improvements in NHS productivity of 2% per annum.

10.2 This means we expect the NHS to match the productivity performance of the wider UK economy. These gains will go back into frontline patient care. Around half of these gains will come from improvements in cost efficiency, which will be delivered by reducing variations in costs between different local health services and by finding new and better ways of working. The remainder will come from improvements in service quality, as the implementation of our reforms raises the standard of patient care.

10.3 The Budget 2002 settlement gives scope for the NHS at a national level to plan ahead with certainty and confidence. With resources being devolved to the local health services they need to share in this certainty. From 2003–04, we intend to maximise the benefits of national level three year expenditure plans by moving to three year revenue and capital allocations to local health services. This will provide a surer foundation for PCTs to plan ahead for improvements in NHS performance.

10.4 The provision of substantial additional resources for the NHS makes improvements in the system of public accountability more necessary. The NHS now needs to more coherently account for how resources have been used and how performance has improved, both nationally and locally.

10.5 In order to ensure clearer public accountability we will strengthen the system of inspection for health and social services. The current system has evolved rapidly. But early experience is demonstrating that the arrangements are fragmented. This is burdensome on front line staff and also creates a lack of clarity for the public. The Bristol Royal Infirmary Inquiry recommended that the number of bodies inspecting and regulating health and social care should be rationalised. The Inquiry also recommended that regulation of the public and private health sectors should be brought together. The Government accepts these recommendations.

10.6 At present the Audit Commission, the National Care Standards Commission and the Commission for Health Improvement (CHI) all play an important and effective role in regulating and assessing healthcare performance. Whilst each has made an important contribution to improving standards, the same local NHS organisation can face multiple uncoordinated visits and demands for information from these and other bodies because of the current fragmentation in the structure of NHS inspection. Fragmentation not only makes for unnecessary bureaucracy, it weakens the system of inspection. It makes for confusion about how well the NHS is performing for those working in the NHS, for patients who use it and for taxpayers who fund it. We now propose radical change.

10.7 We are proposing to establish an independent, single new Commission for Healthcare Audit and Inspection (CHAI) which will bring together the health value for money work of the Audit Commission, the work of the Commission for Health Improvement and the private healthcare role of the National Care Standards Commission. The new single Commission will have responsibility for inspecting both the public and private health care sectors. Its principal roles will include:

- inspecting all NHS hospitals;
- licensing private health care provision;
- conducting NHS value for money audits on a national basis;
- validating published performance assessment statistics on the NHS, including waiting list information;
- publishing star ratings for all NHS organisations with the ability to recommend special measures where there are persistent problems;
- publishing reports on the performance of NHS organisations both individually and collectively;
- independent scrutiny of patient complaints;
- publishing an annual report to Parliament on national progress on health care and how resources have been used.

10.8 New legislation will be needed to establish the Commission. The new Commission will be more independent of Government than the Audit Commission, CHI or the NCSC. Commissioners will be appointed by the Independent Appointments Commission, rather than by Ministers, and in accordance with Nolan rules. The Commissioners, rather than Ministers, will appoint a Chief Inspector of Healthcare.

10.9 The Commission will have the key role in particular in explaining to the public how NHS resources have been deployed and the impact they have had in improving services, raising standards and improving the health of the nation. For the first time the NHS – and indeed private health care – will have a single rigorous inspectorate armed with the ability to expose poor practice and highlight good practice. The new Commission will help strengthen accountability and transparency between the health service and the public who pay for it.

10.10 Similar changes are needed in social services. Here too, there is fragmentation and confusion. The Social Services Inspectorate (SSI) and the National Care Standards Commission both play a role in the inspection of social care services. The SSI is part of the Department of Health with its own Chief Inspector. The NCSC is a non-departmental public body with responsibilities for regulating social care (and private health care) to national standards.

10.11 We now propose to establish a single inspectorate for social services formed from a merger of the two existing organisations. The Commission for Social Care Inspection will:

- carry out local inspections of all social care organisations – public, private and voluntary – including care homes to ensure national standards and publish reports of these inspections;
- register services that meet national standards;
- carry out inspections of local authority social service departments;
- validate all published performance assessment statistics on social care;
- publish the star ratings for social service authorities, with the ability to recommend special measures where there are persistent problems;
- publish an annual report to Parliament on national progress on social care and an analysis of where resources have been used.

10.12 Legislation will be needed to establish the new independent Commission. It will have a key role in driving up standards and strengthening accountability between social services and the public.

10.13 There will be a legal requirement placed on the two new Commissions to co-operate with one another. We have considered the option of establishing a single Commission to cover both services but believe that the organisational upheaval and the extended scope would not be justified. We will, however, keep the situation under review.

10.14 To accompany strengthened accountability at a national level there needs to be strengthened accountability at the local level too. Indeed as power and resources pass down to local health services the requirement to account better to local communities increases. The local NHS needs to be able to demonstrate to the communities it serves how resources have been spent and how performance has improved.

10.15 We propose that each Primary Care Trust will from Autumn 2002 publish an annual patient's prospectus with an A to Z of local health services reporting back to the public in the area it serves. The prospectus will contain detailed information on the performance of the PCT itself and also on each of the main local health care providers including local hospitals. The prospectus will report:

- the assessment the new Commission for Healthcare Audit and Inspection has made of the performance of all major local health care providers;
- an analysis of how each provider has achieved against their previous year's plans and compared to other providers;
- an outline of their next year's plans;
- an analysis of feedback from patients including complaints about each health care provider;
- the results for each local provider of the new system of annual patient surveys, which will form a major plank for measuring the performance of the NHS as a whole;
- a digest of any health inspection reports on any local provider;
- a description of how local health resources were spent last year;
- a plan for how local health resources are to be spent in the coming year.

10.16 This will mean that for the first time, citizens will have independently validated information about how their money has been spent on healthcare in their own area and what progress has been made. The prospectus will outline future plans, and explain how people can get more fully involved if they wish. The prospectus will go to each household in the locality served by the PCT so strengthening the links between the local health service and the local community. Every household in the country will in future know how health service resources have been used and how performance has improved.

10.17 The prospectus will help to inform local communities about standards and services in their area. By doing so they will strengthen local accountability and enhance the Overview and Scrutiny of local health services which from next April will be led by elected local government.

10.18 All patients have a right to expect access to services that are improving, that are free and that are based on their clinical need and their informed choice. But as citizens, we all have a responsibility to ensure that we use health resources fairly and appropriately. So as we improve the rights and experiences of patients, we must do more to strengthen responsibilities.

10.19 We therefore intend to take three further steps on reform here too:

10.20 Firstly, we will do more to protect NHS staff from violent patients. Doctors and nurses are rightly the most highly respected and trusted professionals in the country. Sadly there is a minority of patients who verbally or physically assault NHS staff who are there to help them. We have already made significant progress with our Zero Tolerance policy in acute Trusts. We now must do more to ensure that all GPs also have access to secure services for the treatment of violent patients. We will provide extra resources to PCTs to deal with violent patients. Patients who are persistently violent will find that – subject to appropriate safeguards – they can be denied treatment.

10.21 Secondly, we will do more to reduce the inappropriate use of valuable health care resources. We will start with ambulance services. Some studies of 999 calls to ambulance services have shown that 46% of all callers had medical needs, but did not require an emergency response, and that 12% of callers have no injury or illness at all. Alongside reminding Ambulance Trusts that there is no obligation to attend 999 calls where sending an ambulance is clearly not the best way of helping the patient or using NHS resources, we will back prosecutions against individuals who persistently make hoax calls to the ambulance service.

10.22 Thirdly, to ensure that this agenda begins to take hold in the NHS each PCT will negotiate a new contract on rights and responsibilities through consultation with their communities. The new contract could be agreed upon the point of registration, and form the basis for a mature doctor-patient relationship based on mutual rights and responsibilities.

10.23 Further action will also be examined. As rights grow as services improve so this new agenda of matching patients' rights with responsibilities will be embedded across the NHS.

10.24 Our approach to strengthening the responsibilities of patients and citizens will be evolutionary. We are in the middle of implementing reforms that will significantly improve rights of access to the NHS through booked admissions systems. As waiting times reduce, and rights of access improve, so we will strengthen the responsibilities that we all have to use valuable NHS resources fairly and appropriately. The first phase of our reforms outlined here will help to clarify existing rights and responsibilities, encourage a cultural shift in the way we use finite resources and provide a basis for further development and reform.

11 Conclusion

11.1 The Budget 2002 settlement set out the next steps for investment in the NHS and social care. Alongside the investment must come radical reform. The NHS Plan is and remains the most comprehensive and fundamental package of reforms for the health service since 1948. The NHS Plan is the foundation on which these next steps for reform will be built.

11.2 The NHS now faces a period of unprecedented investment. There can be no excuses for a failure to face up to the radical reforms now necessary.

11.3 Health spending in our country, over the years ahead, will now meet and exceed the European average. Hitting the European average in one year though, will not by itself deliver services equivalent to or better than those of other European countries where high levels of spending have been sustained for years. The only way to ensure that the rising levels of resources unlock rising levels of performance is to fundamentally alter the way health care has been organised, managed and run in our country for half a century.

11.4 There is no automatic correlation that tax-funded health care has to mean health care supply run by Central Government. Other European countries operate tax-funded health systems where decentralisation and choice are essential features. We can learn from them.

11.5 More and more of day-to-day Whitehall control will end. The Department of Health will set standards and put in the resources. Inspection and audit will be independent of the Department. A growing share of a growing NHS budget is being devolved directly to the professionals at the NHS frontline. More investment decisions will be made within the NHS not within Whitehall. And, within the framework of the NHS Plan, there will not be a raft of new targets for the NHS to deliver.

11.6 Power will shift from the centre to the frontline – and flow through to the patient. Since 1948 the NHS has largely been unable to ensure explicit choices for patients. The Government's investment and reforms will make patient choice in the NHS a reality. Heart patients will be the first NHS patients to benefit.

11.7 For more than 50 years the way incentives worked, or didn't work, in the NHS has held back innovation and prevented improvements in performance. The reforms we will now make will ensure that hospitals are paid by results, that the resources for health care go alongside the health care that is delivered. The extra patients who get treated, waiting less time for treatment, will be the main beneficiaries of this reform.

11.8 The reforms we are making will bring health and social care closer together than at any time since the birth of the NHS. Older people and their families will see the benefits for themselves.

11.9 The NHS is now on a stable financial footing to face the future with confidence: with the NHS Plan in place; investment and reforms beginning to show results; power shifting from Whitehall to the NHS frontline. The changes will take time but the benefits for patients are beginning to come through. With this level of investment and commitment to reform the best days of the NHS are ahead of us, not behind us.

Printed in the UK for The Stationery Office Limited
On behalf of the Controller of Her Majesty's Stationery Office
Id 94121 04/02